MW01713211

Ask
Drs. Bob and Elvis

How To
Maintain Your Health

Accessing that Divine Force within us to attain or regain and maintain Divine Health.

Ask
Drs. Bob and Elvis

How To
Maintain Your Health

Accessing that Divine Force within us to attain or regain and maintain Divine Health.

Bob L. Owen, Ph.D., D.Sc., C.R.
Elvis A. Ali, Ph.D., D.Hom., N.D.

HealthHope Books

"My people are destroyed for lack of knowledge" (Hosea 4:6).

The information in this book is based on published and unpublished sources. The purpose is for educational and research purposes only and should not be construed as giving medical advice. The authors and publisher do not diagnose, treat or prescribe. If the reader uses the information to solve his/her own health problems, they are prescribing for themselves, which is their constitutional right, but neither the author nor publisher assume any responsibility.

First printing, August 2001

Library of Congress Control Number: 00-133875
ISNB: 1-882657-20-9
Copyright © 2001 by Bob L. Owen, Ph.D., D.Sc., C.R.
All rights reserved.
Cover Design by Carlo Krouzian

HeathHope Publishing House
10600 Sepulveda Blvd., Suite 102
Mission Hills, CA 91345

To Patricia . . .
Without whose loving encouragement
and endless rereading and
meticulous editing, this book
would never have been completed.
- Dr. Bob . . .

I would like to acknowledge my lovely wife, Khadija and our three children, Hassan, Azeeda and Kareem. They are the most precious gifts I have and they continue to support and motivate me to educate others about naturopathic medicine. My wonderful parents, Hakim and Hazrah along with my sisters, Alima, Homaida (Anna), Homeeda (Lily) and Fazida (Fay) for their support and encouragement, and . . .

Patricia McKenzie, Vice-President, James Maranda, President, Sharon Klinner, Tara Dawn Austin, Teresa Racco, Ken Davrey, Sangeet Sayai, Kim Firth along with the entire Swiss Herbal Remedies staff.

- Dr. Elvis . . .

Foreword

Scripture indicates that humankind is divine, created by God himself and inspired with the breath of life (Genesis 2:7). Along with the divine charge to reproduce, occupy the globe and subdue it, humanity is entrusted with responsibility to preserve the earth and all nature and consume its yield wisely: "I have given you every herb yielding seed, which covers the earth, and every tree which contains the fruit of a tree yielding seed – that shall be your food." (Genesis 1:28-29; 2:15)

The proper care and preservation of our planet can be done only by healthy people – healthy in body, mind and spirit. Physical care of one's being, physical and spiritual are divinely ordained.

Hebrew scriptures, therefore, are filled with the names of many healthful, healing foods to promote health and well-being: "wheat and barley, vines, fig trees and pomegranates, olive oil and honey" (Deuteronomy 8:8), foods that were to be planted and eaten in abundance. These foods were all mentioned and recommended thousands of years ago and recognized today as being totally beneficial to one's health.

Maimonides (1135-1204) the great rabbi, philosopher and physician, wrote extensively on the necessity of maintaining the health of both body and soul, for "the spirit of man is the lamp of the Lord, searching (one's) innermost recesses" Proverbs 20:27).

This book's purpose, therefore, is to provide information, advice and spirituality, the spirituality that imbued "the morning stars (who) sang together, and all the sons of God shouted for joy" (Job 38:4, 6-7) at the divine act of creation. God and Nature, decree that the body dies, decomposes and returns to its primary elements, but the divine soul or intellect, is immortal. Hopefully, this book will provide food for body, mind and spirit, so that we can extend our lives on this earth.

- S. David Garshowitz, B.Sc., Pharm., F.A.C.A., Compounding Pharmacist, integrating mainstream medicine and natural medicine at Yorkdowns Pharmacy, in Toronto, Ontario; Libby Garshowitz, M.A., Ph.D., retired professor and Associate professor of Near and Middle Eastern Civilizations (faculty of Arts and Science of University of Toronto). *-June 19, 2001.*

CONTENTS

Part I

Divine Health: Our Divine Possibility	**9**
Why Are Not All Healed?	**10**
We Are Spiritual Beings (We Are Spirit)	**11**
Spirit Health Principle:	
Healing Begins Within Our Spirit	**12**
Soul/Mind Health Principle:	
Healing Involves Our Mind	***13***
Physical (Body) Health Principle:	
Healing Involves Our Body	***15***

Part II

Two-Pronged Thrust: Faith and Learning	**19**
Healing Principle	**20**
Nutrient Deficiency	**20**
Healing Principle	**21**
Systemic Toxicity	**21**
Healing Principle	**22**
Our Body's Cells	**22**
Our Body's Systems	**23**
Healing Principle	**25**
Nutrient Saturation	**25**
Healing Principle	**26**
Our Body's Most Basic Nutrients	**26**
Healing Principle	**32**
God's Original Nutritional Program	**32**
A Sustainable Nutritional Framework for Today	**32**
Foods To Eat and Foods To Be Avoided	**33**

What About Organic? 36
How Much Should We Eat? 37

Part III

Understanding Digestion 39
The Mouth 40
The Stomach 41
The Small Intestines 42
The Liver/Gallbladder, Pancreas 43
The Pancreas 45
The Kidneys 46
The Large Intestines 46
Systemic Toxicity 47
The Thyroid Gland 48

Part IV

Detoxification 50
The Liver Cleanse 50
The Coffee Enema 53
The Kidney Cleanse 55
Colon Cleansing 58
In A Perfect World . . . 59
Suggested Personal Research Reading 61
Dear Drs. Bob and Elvis . . . 62

Part I

"Beloved, I pray above all things that you may prosper ***and be in health,*** *just as your soul prospers" (The Third Epistle of John, verse 2).*

Divine Health: Our Divine Possibility

IN THE SCRIPTURE above, the Apostle John was speaking of Divine Health, which we believe, even as he does, is our divine possibility. At age 80, Dr. Bob is proving this possibility to be an actuality in his own body, for he is living in divine health, and we believe it possible for every person to do the same.

Which is why we have written this book: fundamentally to help God's people to understand the partnership aspect of healing; consisting of God's part as well as our part. It's not all up to Him. Neither is it all up to us. Faith is involved, of course. But we must educate our *faith-ing*, so we can clearly understand which segment of the healing equation is God's part, and which part is distinctly ours.

For the past decade we have counseled with hundreds of people who were struggling with health issues, many of them full of guilt because they seemed unable to receive the divine health that the Apostle John prayed for all God's people.

Many had prayed and believed for the health and healing the Scriptures promise, that was purchased and paid for by Christ's redemptive work on the cross (Isaiah 53:6), but as the years slipped by and their health continued to decline, they became more and more confused and guilt-ridden . . .

And as health challenges increased their faith has decreased proportionately. All too often their former prayer of faith has become a desperate cry of pain arising from their sick bed:

"Why me, Lord? Why? Why? Why?" To which there seems to be no answer.

So, if you or someone you know is struggling with health Challenges, and the seeming inability to pray "the prayer of faith" that James spoke of (James 5:15), in which "the Lord shall raise him (or you) up," then this book may be for you.

We pray, along with the Apostle John, that you may be *in health,* and that as you read, God will quicken your spirit to hear this word of truth.

And that as you truly hear with ears of faith, may it be with You as it was with the lame man described in Acts 3:7, that your "feet and ankle bones" (along with various other organs and limbs) will begin to receive strength, and your divinely-promised health will begin to materialize.

Beloved, it can be so.

The two distinct purposes of this book are: *First*, to disseminate certain valuable information concerning the processes involved in attaining, regaining, and/or maintaining one's health. The *second,* equally important, is addressed to those who are yearning to be made free from pain, sickness and disease. The two purposes combine to help answer the question below:

Why Are Not All Healed?

This is an honest question that deserves an honest answer. Simply, *it's because those who were, and/or are healed, did not (or do not) understand all that's involved in the healing process.*

Before we proceed, let us make it very clear: We believe that God can heal instantly. He did so in the Biblical era. He still does today. However, all too often, *the healing that was received did (or does) not last.* Why was, or is that still the case?

Basically, we believe it was because the Principles of Healing were not fully understood and followed.

Pain and illness are often "wake-up" calls, by which our Bodies are trying to tell us something in our lifestyle is not conducive to good health. In other words, symptoms indicate a lack of ease; or *dis-ease*. They are communications directly from our magnificently-God-constructed bodies, trying to tell us that something is wrong. If we listen, and hear what our bodies are telling us, and make the necessary "in-flight corrections" to our nutrition and lifestyle, then our 100 trillion or so cells will thank us, and our health will return (or remain).

However, if we (stubbornly or ignorantly) fail to listen to what our bodies are telling us . . . then, trouble and ill health will most certainly eventually manifest.

Three in One: A brief theological statement is in order: the trichotomy of our being. Meaning: The totality of our beings is constructed of three integrally connected, inseparable units: body, soul and spirit. If we are to get a firm grip upon the healing process, and desire to attain, regain or maintain our health, we must understand . . . *We are a spirit; we possess a soul (mind); and we live in a body.*

Read that last statement again if you must, because for us to receive (attain, regain and/or maintain) healing in our physical body, we must cleanse (detoxify) and nourish (feed), our spirits, our souls and our bodies.

Why is that the case? Because, basically, only one or both of two things stand between us and total, divine health:

- toxicity (uncleanness) of spirit, soul or body, and/or,
- adequate nutrition (food) for our spirit, and our soul, and our body.

We Are Spiritual Beings (We Are Spirit)

One merely needs to be present at the moment of death, when the spirit of a man, woman or child departs and is gone from the body, to realize that something intangible has occurred and that the being that remains is spirit-less, and hence life-less.

One cannot dialogue with such a "person," because it contains no living soul (mind) with which to communicate. Synonymous with the human spirit's departure, all evidence of "life" has ceased: cellular generators have shut down and no electrical energy flows; blood no longer circulates; and the body grows cold.

Therefore, life as we understand it, depends upon the residence of a God-given spirit (Living Entity). Such spirit within us *is Life*: the Life Force. Life Energy.

So, if one's spirit and soul are properly cleansed and fed, then all that remains to be done for good health to manifest, is for us to, (a) cleanse our bodies from toxins and negative lifestyles and, (b) provide them with correct quantities of nourishing food.

The inevitable, natural result will be healing.

Spirit Health Principle: Healing Begins within Our Spirit

When one's spirit is in harmony with the Spirit of the living God, *healing power is present*, and it is possible for healing to occur. How does one attain a harmonious relationship with the living God? Through forgiveness: through the *cleansing of our spirit.*

We must see ourselves through God's eyes, and be aware of the things that are an abomination unto Him:

Spirit Toxicity: "A proud look, a lying tongue, hands that shed innocent blood, a heart that devises wicked plans, feet that are swift in running to evil, a false witness who speaks lies, and one who sows discord among brethren" (Proverbs 6:16-19).

How does one receive this forgiveness, this cleansing of the spirit? Simply by asking Him, in all sincerity, to forgive you.

"If we confess our sins (toxicity/filthiness of our human spirit), He is faithful and just to forgive us our sins and to cleanse us from all unrighteousness" (I John 1:9).

Remember: *toxicity*, uncleanness of the spirit, clogs the channels between us and God, making it impossible for us to commune with him, to fellowship with Him.

Forgiveness cleans out the garbage, enabling the free flow of His Spirit between us.

Spirit Nutrition: Once the garbage has been disposed of (cleansing), it is crucial to supply one's spirit with spiritual nourishment: accomplished by spending daily time communing with the Lord; seeking and fellowshiping with others of like mind.

The alternative to spiritual nutrification is unthinkable; which is the point of one of Jesus' parables. "When the unclean spirit (toxic spirit) goes out of a man," Jesus said, "he (the unclean spirit) goes through dry places, seeking rest; and finding none, he says, 'I will return to my house from which I came.'

"And when he comes (returns), he finds it swept and put to order. Then he goes and takes with him seven other spirits more wicked than himself, and they enter and dwell there; and the last state of that man is worse than the first," (Luke 11:24-26).

If you require assistance in finding a "spiritual-nourishment partner," or friend to help show you the way, Jesus reminds us, "Ask, and it (spiritual nourishment) will be given . . . . For everyone who asks receives" (Matthew 7:7-8).

Remember, if we persistently, confidently ask, we *will receive.* Most of us need this kind of assistance. Perhaps your pastor or a teacher can help direct you to a fellowship group of Spirit-filled, Spirit-led people to help guide you, and who will walk a spiritual pathway with you.

Soul/Mind Health Principle: *Healing Involves Our Mind*

The soul or mind of man is the thinking, *knowing part*. It is with the mind that we have the ability to reason and acquire knowledge; the ability to plan; to create and to make decisions. These knowing and reasoning abilities apparently set us apart from the beasts of the field, the fowls of the air, and every living thing on the earth, over which God has charged us with the awesome responsibility of taking dominion (Genesis 1:26, 28).

It is this incredibly creative mind that gives us the power to make choices, to be and become self-determining creatures. It is through our conscious minds that we make the choices that determine our destiny on earth and the hereafter. We have been given the ability to choose our life path; to decide what we want to do or accomplish with our lives.

Within the limits of our culture, we also may choose where we live, the type of work, occupation or profession we desire to follow. And it is with the mind that we make the determination of how well we treat our bodies; how we clothe them, feed them, nurture them or abuse them.

Soul/Mind Toxicity: "I call heaven and earth as witnesses today . . . (says the Lord), that I have set before you life and death, blessing and cursing: *therefore choose life*, that both you and your descendants may live" (Deuteronomy 30:19).

We have been given the power of choice in these matters. What we do with this power is up to us. If we truly desire to *live in divine health*, the power of choice to do so is at our disposal; needing only to be acted upon.

Wrong Thinking and Choices: This power of choice God speaks of in the above Scripture, refers comprehensively with all matters of our thought (soul/mind) life, *right or wrong*. Example: constantly dwelling on negative thoughts; dwelling on fearful thoughts; thoughts of hatred and unforgiveness. All such thoughts deal with death; not with life, and fill our minds (souls) with toxins and poisons, *which must be cleansed away*.

Thus it is within our power, which we can accomplish, by "bringing every thought into captivity," by consciously controlling what goes on in our minds and by resisting everything "that exalts itself against the knowledge of God" (2 Corinthians 10:5).

When we consciously and volitionally do this, we begin the mind-cleansing process.

Mind Nutrition: It is then and only then, as we "receive with meekness the implanted word" (James 1:21), that the mind-nourishment process begins, by providing "food (nutrition) for our soul."

But, how do we go about "transforming" and "renewing" our minds?

Again, *we accomplish this, by obeying God's command*: "Do not be conformed to this world, but be transformed by the renewing of your mind (a conscious act of will), that you may prove what is that good and acceptable and perfect will of God" (Romans 12:2). It is *with our m*inds that we reason. It is *with our minds* that we select and *make the choices* that determine, not only our eternal destiny, but the health and physical well being of our finite bodies.

We transform and renew ourselves by allowing God's words to fill our minds; by cherishing His words (His Word) in our heart; by thinking His thoughts. When we begin to do this, it is then that His concepts will lead us while we are awake. And even when we sleep, His thoughts will permeate our dreams (Proverbs 6:21-22).

It is through this "attending to God's words" that spiritual (soul/mind) healing begins to manifest itself. For when the mind is filled with healing/nutritional thoughts, there is no remaining room for toxic thoughts to penetrate; thus preventing a "toxic buildup" of negativity, fear and other mind-poisoning thoughts.

"Consent and submit to my sayings," (He says to us). "Let them (His words) not depart from your sight; keep them in the center of your heart. For they (God's healing words) are life to those who find them (and incorporate them into their minds), healing and health to all their flesh" (Proverbs 4:20-22, *Amplified Bible*).

God never commands us to do something we are not capable of doing. Resources are always available, if we will only deliberately fix our minds and thoughts upon Him: "Finally, brethren, whatever things are true, whatever things are noble, whatever things are just, whatever things are pure, whatever things are lovely, whatever things are of good report, if there is any virtue and if there is anything praiseworthy, meditate (think) on these things" (Philippians 4:8).

Physical (Body) Health Principle: *Healing Involves Our Body*

This temple of flesh and blood (our body) provides housing for our spirit and soul (mind); although both our spirits and souls can soar beyond the finite limitations of our bodies. Our bodies, however, are somewhat firmly fixed upon the Earth.

Few would doubt that life itself, in all its ramifications, is a gift of God. Not every one, however agrees as to how we should deal with, and/or feed, house and clothe our physical bodies; and some eat and drink without ever consulting God for His wisdom and direction concerning the nurturing of His temple.

"I beseech you therefore, brethren, by the mercies of God, that you present your bodies a living sacrifice, holy, acceptable to God, which is your reasonable service" (Romans 12:1).

Physical (Body) Toxicity: Thus, many people tend to treat their bodies as though nothing can harm them; often making poor or detrimental food choices; choosing abusive lifestyles that eventually brings harm to their bodies, lessening the quality of their lives and frequently shortening their existence.

These poor or detrimental food choices and abusive lifestyles are toxic (poisonous) to our bodies.

An overload of toxic substances in our bodies can make us sick. It can also cause serious pain. Not counting the pain associated with accidental injuries such as those suffered in accidents, or a critical disease, or the pain of childbirth (a category by itself), most chronic pain is caused by a toxic condition.

Pain and disease are nature's effort to eliminate toxins from the blood. Therefore, in actuality, most so-called diseases are simply crises of toxemia or toxic poisoning.

Does Eliminating Pain Eliminate the Disease?

Much of current medical philosophy focuses on "treating" pain with drugs. In many cases drugs quickly help eliminate the pain, usually quite effectively.

But does it cure the disease or problem?

No. It merely masks the pain.

But the cause of the pain remains.

Unless **the cause of the pain** is eliminated, the problem will remain and become worse, finally resulting in tissue and organ failure or breakdown and eventually a so-called "degenerative" disease, such as diabetes, heart disease, arthritis, cancer, or another serious, often fatal disease.

The only way to effectively eliminate pain is to remove the cause. This may take time: weeks, months, and often years.

Why do doctors prescribe and patients take, and continue to take drugs?

It's because treating the pain with drugs is usually simple and quick, giving one a false sense of security. With pain artificially removed (even for a few minutes or days), one is tempted to think that he or she is healed. But, in every case, unless the cause of the pain has been eliminated, the pain-causing problem simply "goes underground" and continues to proliferate.

It will eventually surprise us by "suddenly" overtaking us in a way and to such a degree that the drugs will no longer work.

At such a time drastic means are often employed: usually surgery, chemotherapy or radiation.

How does one go about discovering and removing the cause of the pain? Or, to ask the question in a different way: How does one attain or maintain a healthy body?

Very simply stated, it is by choosing to obey God's laws of sowing and reaping.

And, that's what this book is all about.

In the majority of cases, citizens of America (and much of the developing world) have not been taught how to care for their bodies in such a way as to prevent toxicity and subsequent sickness. As a consequence, many, by intent or simply because of failure to properly care for their bodies, find themselves in pain with their bodies beginning to deteriorate; then frantically begin seeking for a healer to help them reverse the process of degeneration that is hastening them toward an untimely death.

We must realize that we "are the temple of God" and that His Spirit dwells in us. We must also recognize that if we defile this temple, we will destroy it. Perhaps, to be more accurate, the defiling of this temple will result in the physiological degeneration of our bodies.

How does one defile a temple or a house? Or a body? One way is to despoil it with loads of garbage.

How does one "undefile" a temple or a house? Or a body? By cleaning out the debris, and preventing more of the same from coming in.

Physical (Body) Nutrition: How does one care for his or her temple? By learning how your body functions. How to do this? Select books from "Suggested Reading" on the last page of this book. Make yourself responsible for your own health. Ask God to direct you to a health professional you can trust. Form a partnership with that person, with the goal of learning how to care for and (nutritionally) feed your body.

Why? Because our body is the temple of God and a visible reflection (example) of health (or lack of health).

Every individual body is different. But the principles of caring for all bodies are the same: TLC (tender loving care).

It seems abundantly clear that if we are to attain, regain and/or maintain divine health, we must willingly offer our bodies to God, along with the entirety of our triune beings. Along with the offering of both our spirit life and soul life (minds) to Him, *it is the final and complete offering to Him — "that you present your bodies a living sacrifice, holy, acceptable unto God . . . (our) reasonable service" (Romans 12:1), that completes the transaction,* making it possible for us to walk and live in divine health.

PART II

Wisdom is the principal thing; Therefore, get wisdom. And in all your getting, get understanding (Proverbs 4:5, 7).

This section focuses on acquiring the knowledge to take personal responsibility for one's own health and *learning how* to cleanse (detoxify) and nurture (feed) our physical beings.

Two-Pronged Thrust: Faith and Learning

Faith plays a prominent role in receiving anything from God, including forgiveness from sin for the spirit, cleansing of the mind (soul) or physical healing of the body. "For without faith it is impossible to please Him (God), for he who comes to God must believe that He is, and that He is a rewarder (will answer your prayers) of those who diligently seek Him" (Hebrews 11:6).

Doctors often speak of the "placebo effect," which greatly determines the effectiveness of any medication or treatment. For example, if a person does not believe that a drug or medication will (or might) work for him, in most cases it won't. On the other hand, even if the doctor gives a patient a sugar pill with the admonition that it will cure their problem or disease; if the patient has faith in the doctor and believes he has been told the truth, then, in spite of the medication, or whatever he has been told to do or to take, his condition will improve or be healed.

Faith, of course, is required of one if he or she is to please God. And, as God repeatedly shows us, *Faith is closely allied with learning.* We are to improve our faith, with study; by educating ourselves. "Study to show yourself approved unto God, a workman that needeth not to be ashamed, rightly dividing the word of truth (knowledge)" (2 Timothy 2:15). This includes matters of health.

Together, faith and personal effort focused on a goal, form a dynamic duo that God will bless, and guide us into the truth of health and healing. In the light of this fact, several Healing Principles apply that will enable us to more clearly see God's hand in our healing potential.

Healing Principle

Growing numbers of health professionals believe *the most difficult, intractable diseases have only two causes: nutrition deficiency and/or systemic toxicity*. Both must be remedied as quickly as possible, or decreased levels of health will manifest.

Nutrition Deficiency

The first culprit is probably the worst: **nutrition deficiency**, sometimes called under-nutrition, or malnutrition. Presently there are approximately 50 factors that are *essential to life*, of which 45 are nutrients. In this context, *essential* is defined as something the body needs, cannot make for itself, but must be obtained from the environment.

If each and every one of these nutrients is essential – meaning the body cannot get along without them – to the health and well-being of our bodies, it's only reasonable to assume that the lack (deficiency) of any one or more of such nutrients would result in the weakening or malfunction of certain body tissues or organs.

That's exactly what happens. For example, since bones and teeth are manufactured primarily from calcium, if our bodies were lacking in calcium, our bones and teeth would not develop properly. And since, among other nutrients, our heart muscles must be assured of an adequate supply of magnesium to function properly, the lack of that essential nutrient is bound to result in some kind of heart malfunctioning.

Likewise, an imbalance of sodium and potassium at the cellular level, will cripple the proper functioning of the body's vital electrical generators that are responsible for creating energy.

Hence, the seriousness of nutrient deficiency, which is the all-important, underlying hidden predisposing first cause for illness of any kind. I call it the Nutrient Deficiency Syndrome (NDS), that works in our bodies by setting the stage, preparing the ground, and acting behind the scenes, painlessly, silently and treacherously bringing about poor health and disease.

More than any other single cause Nutritional Deficiency Syndrome (NDS) illustrates the seriousness of improper nutrition and helps illustrate the fundamental reasons for the development of cancer and AIDS, heart and kidney disease, arthritis, Alzheimer's disease and strokes, osteoporosis, premature aging and other degenerative conditions.

The principles are the same: If we don't properly and consistently feed our spirit and mind, spiritual (soul/mind) nutritional deficiencies can accrue. If or when that happens, spiritual toxicity (poisoned thinking) may begin to invade our thoughts; even as toxicity invades our bodies when they become nutritionally deficient.

Healing Principle

If the body is adequately supplied with all necessary nutrients, our immune systems will be strong and healthy, and able to ward off any foreign invaders.

Systemic Toxicity

The second, more visible "cause" of disease-toxicity can come about only if one's body is nutrient deficient. I call this **systemic toxicity**. Simply stated, systemic toxicity means our entire system (the whole body) is loaded with uneliminated toxins or poisons.

These poisons make the cells sick. Sick cells become sick tissues. Sick tissues make up the organs, which also become sick. Reasonably, then, when we have sick cells, sick tissues and sick organs, the entire body (system) is sick, to a lesser or greater degree, depending upon the amount and kinds of toxins in the body.

What Are These Toxins?

Toxic substances are recognized publicly by such terms as *asbestos, bacteria, carcinogens (cancer-producing substances) of all kinds, cholesterol, overuse of drugs, food dyes and additives, fungus, pesticides and herbicides, lead paint, polluted air, water and food, tobacco smoke and X-rays,* ***to name a few***. This is a short list of the various substances and means by which our bodies can become poisoned and re-poisoned by toxins that we are unable to eliminate.

It must be understood that toxicity (poisonous matter in the body) must be removed as quickly as possible or decreased levels of health will soon result. Tachycardia (increased heart rate), for example, indicates that some form of toxicity is present.

Healing Principle

Bodies that are saturated with essential nutrients are generally able to eliminate toxins almost as quickly as they enter, making a maximally nutrified person practically invulnerable to sickness.

Remember: Polluted Immune Systems are not strong enough to fight off all the toxins with which they are surrounded every single day of our lives.

Added to the usual toxins to be found in food, air, water and other parts of our environment are yet another: stress. Stresses of any kind – fear, anger, frustration, emotional upsets, as well as hatred, unforgiveness, etc. – acts as a tourniquet around our blood vessels and nerve supply, cutting off or diminishing the flow of proper nutrients to our brain and all other organs. Unrecognized or ignored, stresses of life are hazardous to our Immune Systems.

However, as stated above, if our bodies are nutritionally saturated **and** clean of stored, uneliminated toxins, including stresses, then we should be living in reasonably good health.

How can we best accomplish such a condition?

In a phrase: **By educating ourselves.** By gaining an understanding of the principles of physical health; by learning something of physiology, of how our body operates, and then applying what we learn to our daily lives.

Our Body's Cells

The basic unit of our bodies is the cell: There are approximately 100 trillion of these incredibly complex and complete entities. All of the body's tissues, organs and body systems are composed of cells. Each cell is a self-contained energy unit; a city unto itself, with its own power plant (generator); its own energy distribution center; its own garbage disposal system. Literally everything that happens in the body begins here. Each cell is an electrical generator; and each **healthy cell** constantly and continuously produces an average of 65 millivolts of electricity.

This electrical output is our Life Force and must be maintained at all times. When cells cease producing electrical energy, they die. As cells die (which happens continuously) and are not replaced by new, vital, living cells, our body dies.

Each cell shares the concern and responsibility for keeping us healthy. Each cell in our body, to a certain degree, is autonomous, having the ability to control itself. Recent research has uncovered (or discovered) the immense intelligence and complexity of the cell. It boggles the mind to realize that each cell is operated like a modern, state-of-the-art factory.

In order to keep each of our untold trillions of cells operating efficiently, we must provide them with the resources to feed themselves, digest and assimilate their food, and dispose of the excreted waste. In other words, each cell generally conducts its cycle of life in much the same manner that we do, though on a much smaller, though not less complex operation.

If we are to attain, regain and/or maintain healthy physical bodies, our primary and ongoing responsibility to our body's vast numbers of living cells is to keep them cleansed of toxic materials and to supply them with adequate nutrition.

Our Body's Systems

Our bodies possess many systems, all of them charged with the task of keeping us well. What are they, and what do they do?

- **The Respiratory System** is concerned with the health and well being of our body concerning disease conditions ranging from colds to pneumonia, asthma and allergies and emphysema, among others.
- **The Cardiovascular System** is concerned with the heart, the arteries and veins, blood pressure and disease conditions such as heart attacks, stroke and blood clotting.

- **The Gastrointestinal System (GI System)**, is responsible for the digestion and assimilation of food and the production of energy from that food; and is concerned with such organs as the mouth, esophagus, stomach, liver and gallbladder, pancreas and both the small and large intestine.
- **The Genitourinary System**, covers such organs as the kidneys, prostate, bladder, uterus and ovaries, having a multiplicity of functions.
- **The Musculoskeletal System**: covers all of the bones, muscles, tendons of the body; concerned with the framework that protects our internal organs, the muscles and tendons that enable us to move, as well as protection of the entire body against disease processes that affect these organs, such as arthritis, spinal problems, broken bones, etc.
- **The Endocrine System** deals with the functioning and or malfunctioning of the endocrine glands, namely: pineal gland, pituitary gland, hypothalamus gland, thyroid and parathyroid glands, thymus gland, adrenal glands and kidneys, pancreas, ovaries (female) and testes (male).
- **The Nervous System** that deals with the brain and spinal nerves, along with the body's entire system of nerves; this system is concerned with disease conditions ranging from stroke, Parkinson's disease, Alzheimer's disease, multiple sclerosis, depressions schizophrenia, and related conditions.
- **The Immune System** is not simply an organized group of organs possessing the sole purpose or responsibility of preventing us from becoming ill. Instead, our Immune System is composed of every single cell in our bodies. This means that any time we feel unusually weak, tired and lacking in energy, our body (Immune System) is telling us something is not right and that it's our responsibility to correct it with detoxification, nutrition or rest.

Healing Principle

Because of the way God has designed us, a strong, intact Immune System will make you practically invulnerable to attack from nearly any force (bacterial, viral, fungal [yeast], toxic, pathogenic, emotional, etc.) from within or without.

Nutrient Saturation

While researching another book, Dr. Bob spent some time in a hospital that deals primarily with cancer. Every day the cancer patients would gather for an educational lecture on the causes of the disease that was killing them, and to explore ways and means to become well again.

After the lecture, a patient asked the speaker, "What is the best way to prevent cancer? And, once you have the disease, what's the best way to overcome it, to heal it?"

Without hesitation the speaker said, "Fortify the host."

"Fortify the host? I don't understand," the questioner answered. "What do you mean, 'fortify the host'?"

"*Well*," the lecturer said, "*there are two theories that attempt to explain the cause and cure of all disease, including cancer. The first believes that it's the irresistible attack from outside forces that makes us sick. These people fight force with force, employing even stronger outside forces to kill the invaders.*

"The second theory is based on a totally different philosophy, which is this: *If we keep our bodies well and strong, these strong outside invaders (forces) will be unable to break through our shield of immunity and make us sick.*

"*Personally, I subscribe to the second theory, which makes each of us carry some responsibility for what happens to our own health.*

"*In other words, I believe most bodies become ill because the host – allowed their body to become nutrient deficient, and/or engaged in certain abusive practices. This resulted in their body becoming so overloaded with uneliminated toxins (poisons), that their body broke down and became sick.*"

He paused for emphasis.

"But, if you fortify the host (your body), by keeping it nutritionally saturated, you won't become sick because your strengthened Immune System will keep you well."

I believe that doctor was right.

A weakened or compromised Immune System leaves the door wide open – with the welcome mat prominently displayed – for any and all disease conditions that might be in the neighborhood (water, air, food, soil, textiles, thoughts, emotions, etc.), including such conditions as the so-called "Hong Kong Flu."

Although this principle needs little elaboration, one point is in order: If you desire good health, you and only you are ultimately responsible to see to it that your spirit, soul (mind) and body are kept **nutritionally saturated** at all times. To do less than this is to invite sickness and disease.

Healing Principle

In His wisdom, God has made us responsible for maintaining our own health. Which means that *only you* can keep your Immune System in good condition. It does not happen automatically. And it requires consistent cleansing of spirit, soul (mind) and body, and a consistency in supplying your body with the necessary nutrients.

Our Body's Most Basic Nutrients

There are 4 of them. They are God's gift to us. "In the beginning God created . . ." He created every living thing that we see today, including **Sunlight, Water, Air (Oxygen),** and our bodies. Then He **Rest**ed. Light, Water, Air and Rest. These four elements are the Foundational Factors in our Nutrition Program. They are all crucial to our health. And they cost us nothing – except a minimum amount of effort.

Figure 1 below graphically illustrates the vital underlying importance of these Foundational Factors in providing support to the life-giving nutrition our bodies require.

Air (Oxygen)

Air (oxygen) is the most vital, life-sustaining component in our bodies. During God's creative process, the first man, became a living being when God "breathed into his nostrils the breath of Life." Air (oxygen) is essential for life. We can live for days or

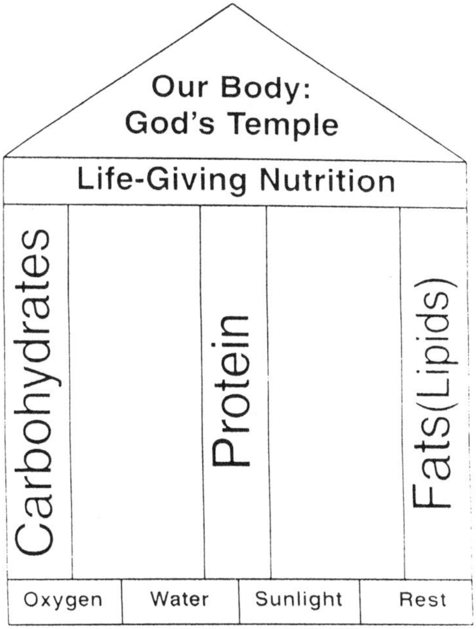

Figure 1: Without the support of the Foundational Factors of Air, Water, Sunlight and Rest, the potential benefits of all the other nutritional factors will be diluted and less beneficial.

weeks without food. We çan live for several days without water. But we can live for only a few minutes without air (oxygen).

Spending a few minutes deep breathing several times a day is essential if we are to supply our 100 trillion cells with oxygen; which is necessary if we are to provide them with sufficient oxygen to continuously produce the mandatory 65 millivolts in the mitochondrian in each cell. This electricity is life itself. When this electricity gets low, our energy gets lower and lower. The lower the electrical generation becomes, the weaker and sicker we become. When our cells are unable to generate electricity, our energy grinds to a halt and stops. Runs down. Then we die. Nothing takes the place of air that's as fresh and clean as possible.

When should we spend time to focus on breathing? Of course, it can be done almost anytime. However, one of the best times may be the first thing in the morning, before we begin to get bogged down with the sheer business of living. Step outside into the freshest air of the day, and breathe . . . exhale. Breathe . . . exhale. Again and again. You will soon notice the benefits of allowing God's fresh air to provide your body with healing oxygen.

Therapeutic breathing works effectively to help calm troubled moods. In fact, taking several deep, slow breaths, drawing air into the lungs and deep into the body, and expanding the abdomen, can have a major impact on feelings of anxiety and upsets. Deep breathing also assists the lungs in their detoxification function. (See Detoxification, pages 50-58.)

Water

Our bodies are approximately 75% water. Our cells are filled with water. Our cells are surrounded with water. Our brain is more than 75% water. The joints between our bones are filled with water. Our muscles are mostly water. Our need for water is second only to oxygen. A mere 20% deficiency is life threatening.

By itself, water is the most healing fluid, the most beneficial medicine, and it is vital to our health. Without water we soon become dehydrated, weak and sickly, diseased and die. "Chronic cellular dehydration," writes Dr. Batmanghelidj, "painfully and prematurely kills. Its initial outward manifestations have until now been labeled as diseases of unknown origin. . . (but) chronic and persistently increasing dehydration is the *root cause* of almost all currently encountered major diseases of the human body." (*Your Bodies Many Cries for Water*, F. Batmanghelidj, M.D.)

Plain, pure water is what our bodies crave. A minimum of several quarts a day. A good rule of thumb is ½ ounce of water per day per pound of weight. Which means, for example, that a man weighing 150 pounds would require a minimum of 75 ounces of this most important life-giving substance, each day. Herbal teas are of secondary importance, but liquids other than water serve to dehydrate. Tea, coffee, juices and other fluids do not count for water and will further dehydrate the body. **Only water hydrates the body and fulfills the body's need for liquids.**

Most health professionals recommend that you *do not drink tap water*, which is almost universally polluted to some degree, and that you choose purified water of some kind. There are many kinds, degrees and varieties of purified water, from a simple carbon filter (which must be changed regularly or it becomes clogged with debris and worse than before); to more sophisticated filtering involving a several-step processes (again, attention must be focused on systematically replacing the filters); to reverse osmosis (an excellent system, but one that reportedly wastes a good deal of water); and distillation (the only method that removes the water from the contaminants, rather than the contaminants from the water.

Many Scriptures, such as Isaiah 55 speak of water as the healing essense of life. "Ho! Everyone who thirsts, Come to the waters." And Jesus Himself emphasizes this analogy: "If anyone thirsts, let him come to Me and drink. He who believes in Me . . . out of his heart will flow rivers of living water" (John 7:37-38).

Sunlight

God's first recorded words referred to light. During His act of Creation, God said, "Let there be light . . ." It is a medical fact that sunlight is crucial to our health. For example: sun-on-skin exposure for as little as 15 minutes a day enables our bodies to produce vitamin D. If our bodies did not receive vitamin D from the sun, calcium, necessary for normal bone growth and development, would not be absorbed from the intestinal tract, and our bones would become deformed.

Whether we live in the north or south, and the day brings us full sun or cloud-covered skies, it is necessary to our health that we spend some time exposing face, arms or body to the sun's healing rays. These health-giving benefits will accrue to us even on days when the sun's face is hidden behind clouds. And, on sun-bright days, we can even benefit from "open shade" exposure.

Figure 2 below illustrates the vital relationship between the sun and the production of vitamin D.

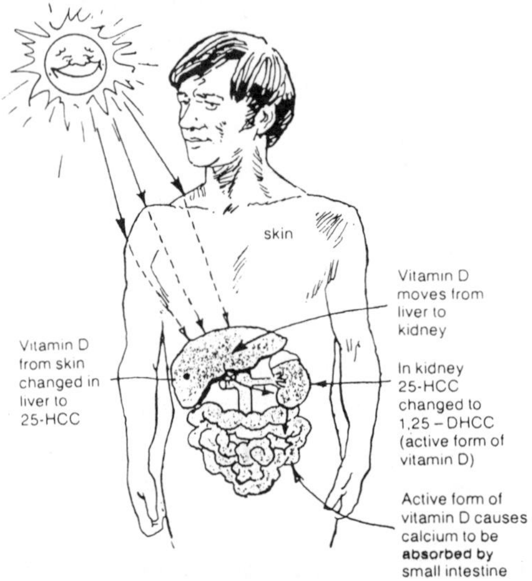

Figure 2. Through an intricate process, sun-on-skin exposure to the sun's rays creates the vitamin D necessary calcium assimilation.

Rest and Sleep

It is not incidental that God concluded the Creation of the Universe with rest, because He knew that rest and sleep are vital to our health and well-being. ***It is only when our bodies are fully relaxed, as in meditation or rest or sleep that our bodies are able to rebuild themselves.*** In today's frenetic, almost non-stop activity, it is small wonder that stress is involved as an element in every disease state. Jesus Himself took time to remove Himself from stressful activities to be alone and rest. For us to fail to build into our schedules regular times of rest is to invite (dis-ease) disease.

A missing ingredient to a person's health may be "Vitamin Zzzzz." Sleep researcher Michael Irwin, M.D. learned that when participants of one study were cheated out of four hours of sleep for four consecutive nights that they had an average of 30% drop in their immune response. This was measured by the person's natural killer-cell activity. Dr. Irwin indicated that such a drop can readily increase one's susceptibility to colds and flu, and perhaps to other serious diseases.

Exercise

In addition to these five Foundational Factors in our Nutrition Program, is the fact that it makes good sense for us to keep our bodies in good physical condition by also taking time to exercise. Our bodies were made to move. Without movement our muscles become stiff and hard; the cells of our lungs cannot expand to draw air and oxygen into our bodies. Our heart becomes weak and cannot pump blood to our extremities. Our arteries get stiff and hard (hardening of the arteries); causing high blood pressure. Without movement, our lymph fluids cannot remove the poisons and toxin from our cells; they become weak and sick and soon die. Persons who lie in bed for days or weeks at a time develop pneumonia because only movement will remove poisons from our lungs.

How much exercise is necessary? Daily stretching is mandatory, which helps keep your muscles and joints limber. Beyond that, the best exercise is brisk walking for 15-30 minutes 3-5 days a week. Bouncing on a mini-trampoline or rebounder for several minutes a day is wonderful; it gets the lymph moving and helps remove toxins from tissues and blood. And practically everyone can do this, no matter what their present physical condition, to help prevent bone loss. The most effective exercise is some form of weight-bearing exercise, especially one that you enjoy and will do consistently.

Along with the daily stretching of our muscles, it's also important to "exercise" one's lungs to provide our cells with sufficient oxygen. This can be accomplished by repeatedly blowing up a rubber balloon. Perhaps difficult at first, after a few days, it will become easier and easier to do. As simple an exercise as this appears to be, you will soon notice that your lung capacity is increasing, making it easier for you to walk and even climb stairs with less effort than before.

Healing Principle

Included in God's Acts of Creation was His varied provision for our nutritional sustenance. Because, *it is the variety of foods that we eat – and assimilate* – that provide us with the nutrients our bodies require, and that will assist our Immune System attain and maintain a sustainable level of health.

God's Original Nutritional Program

God has thought of everything. In His wisdom, God has already provided for all our basic needs, even provision for the foods we need. When He created Adam and Eve, He blessed them with a lovely garden: the Garden in Eden. He showed them what He had done, and told them, "I give you every seed-bearing plant on the face of the whole earth and every tree that has fruit with seed in it. They will be yours for food" (Genesis 1:29, NIV).

Later, God spoke to Noah and his sons, telling them, "Every creature that moves along the ground, and upon all the fish of the sea; they are given into your hands. Everything that lives and moves will be food for you. Just as I gave you the green plants, I now give you everything" (Genesis 9:2-3, NIV).

But, nowhere did God ever mention artificial fertilizers, herbicides, pesticides, genetic modification of plants and meats, or the over-processed convenience foods that we now consume.

He provided mankind with pure, uncontaminated food, air and water, all of which man has polluted to the point that it's becoming more and more difficult to obtain the nutritious, uncontaminated foods and water necessary to sustain health. This situation has resulted in millions of people with impaired health and compromised Immune Systems. Therefore, it has become necessary to devise nutritional programs to help everyone attain, regain, and/or maintain an optimum level of health. The following nutritional program suggests the framework for such an overall plan.

A Sustainable Nutritional Framework for Today

In keeping with God's Original Nutritional Program, the nutritional framework outlined below is designed to assist one's body to create and maintain a vitally necessary level of "balanced body chemistry." This framework can be used with benefit by anyone, **especially those with health challenges.**

The longer you stay with these diet principles and the more closely you follow them, the easier it will be to stick with them, and you will soon find yourself looking and feeling so much better than you did with your old way of eating. As you become healthier, your cravings for ***foods, which are not best choices for you, will actually diminish***. Since old habits are difficult to break or change, take your time in changing your diet habits so you won't quickly fail and slip back into your old ways of eating. Remember: Nutritional supplements may be needed to assist you in getting and staying "on track."

Foods To Eat And Foods To Be Avoided

Proteins: Eat small amounts frequently; preferably a ***small amount*** with each meal. Small is defined as 2-4 ounces of meat, fish, fowl or eggs at any one time. Both animal and vegetarian sources of protein are beneficial. As much as possible, select the healthiest options available: free range, antibiotic free and/or organic. For most people **whole eggs** are an excellent source of protein. Your body needs and uses the lecithin in the yolk to lower blood fat and improve liver and brain function. Grilled, boiled, steamed, soft-boiled or poached are best preparation methods for preparing protein.

Carbohydrates: The eating of carbohydrates tends to become complicated. There are really 3 different kinds of carbohydrates: simple, complex and processed. For anyone with a health challenge, most carbohydrates are off limits. Why? Because the more carbs you eat, the more you crave and *craving carbohydrates is an indication of imbalance*. Principle: Eat vegetables as your primary carbohydrate choice.

Vegetables: Eat more, <u>*more*</u>, ***more*** **VEGETABLES!** Most people with health challenges can greatly improve their health just by doing this. Choose a selection of vegetables. Make the green leafy your preference; such as spinach, chard, beet greens, kale, broccoli, mustard greens, etc.; avoiding iceberg lettuce if possible; rather choosing lettuces with a rich, green color, along with sprouts and raw nuts. Fresh, raw and organic (if possible) is best. Raw is the best preparation method, with lightly steamed, or sautéed as second choice. Use only butter or olive oil for sauté. And, don't make salads your only veggies.

Fruits are also very important. Whole fruit is preferred to juices, which is loaded with simple sugars, which quickly converts to triglycerides and is stored as fat. When eating fruit, it's best to eat only one kind at a time. If your health is not up to par, try to avoid the sweetest fruits (especially tropical fruits), except papaya and pineapple, which are very rich in digestive enzymes.

Grains could be a rich source of vitamins and minerals, if it were not for soil depletion and genetically engineered grains, which now have 5 times the gluten and 1/3, the protein of original wheat. This fact alone accounts for many allergic reactions. Even whole grains can cause trouble. If you do eat them, do so in moderation, and only at dinner. It would be wise to limit even whole grains, and probably best to minimize wheat and barley, replacing them with unprocessed rye, rolled oats and brown rice (white rice has been stripped of nutrients.) Some Danish and German brown breads like pumpernickel, may be a nutritious substitute.

Avoid white flour, which means donuts, muffins, cookies, candies, crackers, pastas, and most bakery goods. These processed carbohydrates are frequently connected with weight gain, heart disease and cancer.

Sugar and other sweeteners: To protect your family health, you would be wise to avoid using Nutra Sweet and other artificial sweeteners, as well as corn syrup and table sugar; from which all the nutrients have been refined out. **Raw** cane sugar, however, does provide some nutrients to aid in its metabolism.

Sugars are a ready source of quick, but short-lasting energy, and should be used in **limited amounts**.

Best sweeteners include raw, unfiltered honey, date sugar granules, pure maple sugar, unsulfured molasses and stevia (which does not affect blood sugar levels). Note: When raw products are stored they tend to harbor molds, which were not destroyed with cooking or pasteurization; and which can be negated by sprinkling a small amount [1/4 teaspoon] of vitamin C in the container before using it, which will protect you without affecting the taste.

Fats and Oils: The good news about Fats and Oils is that small amounts of the right kind of fats and oils are vital to life and health. The bad news is that most people consume too many of the bad kinds and don't get enough of the right kinds. Fats are required for energy, for building cellular membranes and forming hormones. Best are organic, cold-pressed, extra virgin olive oil, walnut oil, flax seed and grape seed oil. Raw butter and olive oil are safe to cook with.

Avoid all hydrogenated and partially hydrogenated fats, as well as "fat-reduced" foods; especially those encouraging you to "eat what (and all) you want, because your body won't absorb it." All such fake foods are poison to your system. Never eat margarine again, as well as all supermarket oils in plain (clear) bottles. Vegetable oils are extremely sensitive to oxygen, heat and sunlight, which degrade the oils, making them tasteless, odorless and worthless. Good oils will have a pleasant nutty taste and aroma.

Eat all the avocados and raw nuts you desire. The right kind of fat is vital to digestion, and **doesn't make you fat!** Fatty fish and/or fish oil is beneficial. Eating "fat-free" products and "low fats" usually means high sugar/high calories; and usually results in consuming more calories than that in un-reduced fat content food. ***Some of the sickest people are those who have been on a fat-free diet for a long time.***

Milk Products: This is a complex, controversial subject. Although pasteurization diminishes the total value of milk, including its mineral, vitamin B and calcium content, ***milk is still probably the best, most assimilable source of calcium***, but it must be 2% or higher in butter fat to be effective. On the other hand, the vitamins and minerals and trace minerals in raw milk (though it is difficult to obtain in most areas) are 100% available. The public has been advised that raw milk may not be safe. Raw milk dairies are tested *daily* by an independent laboratory for bacteria, whereas pasteurized milk is tested only 8 times per year by the health department; and the allowable bacterial count in pasteurized milk is somewhat higher than that of raw milk. The primary advantage of pasteurized milk is for the seller's benefit, because pasteurization lengthens the shelf life of the milk. And ultra-pasteurization extends milk's shelf life even further.

Homogenized milk is less digestible. In the homogenation of milk, the size of the fat particles is reduced, permitting them to be assimilated into the bloodstream; which may account (at least in part) to allergies and frequent sinus congestion, especially in children, and the escalating problems associated with clogged blood vessels and heart and circulatory conditions among adults.

In light of the above information, if you are unable to obtain raw milk, limiting or avoiding dairy may make it easier to attain your optimal level of health and hormonal balance. Raw goat and sheep products are great alternatives, because their genetic code and fat content are apparently more like humans. Even so, be careful and use in moderation. Raw butter and Kefir (liquid, **unsweetened** yogurt) are excellent sources of essential nutrients and vitamins. Sweetened yogurt has become increasingly popular, but is loaded with sugar. What about soymilk and rice milk to replace dairy? They sound like healthy alternatives; but are really highly processed simple carbohydrates.

What About Organic?

Foods (and supplements) should be taken in their whole form wherever possible. This applies to all foods, including organic produce. Studies comparing organic to commercial produce have found that commercially grown fruits and vegetables are nutrient poor compared to organic produce. Moreover, commercial produce contains higher amounts of heavy metals than organic foods, most likely as a result of the pesticides and commercial fertilizers used to enhance their growth.

According to research done by the U.S. Organic Association . . .

- Children receive up to 35% of their entire lifetime dose of cancer-causing pesticides by the age of five.
- Trace amounts of 17 pesticides were found in the top baby food sold in the United States.
- Harmful estrogens linked to cancer are found in pesticides.
- 80 % of all cancers are caused by toxic agents in our environment: air, water, food, etc.

It is true that organically grown produce is more expensive than commercially grown produce. And it may not be possible for families to afford higher costing food. But, wherever and whenever possible do so, the difference in quality may be worth it.

Actually, organic food is a great bargain. While the shelf life is often shorter than similar-appearing food grown in the chemical-intensive method, many hidden bonuses come along with the purchase price. The methods used to grow organic food builds our precious soil instead of depleting it, resulting in clear instead of polluted runoff water, preserves the health of farm workers and their children, contributes to the health of the people who eat the food instead of threatening that health with dangerous synthetic chemicals, and helps keep alive the traditional seed varieties that are the foundation of all of humanity's food supply. To receive all of this extra benefit is a greater bargain than most people realize.

How Much Should We Eat?

The answer is: much less than most of us do eat. Digesting food demands a great deal of energy from our bodies. Eating a smaller amount reduces the stress of digestion on our energy supply, and gives our energy generator a chance to keep up by not overwhelming it with a large meal. The average mealtime in the United States is 15 minutes, compared with 1-1/2 hours in Europe. Small wonder Americans suffer from such a high rate of digestive disorders. When digestion is impaired, yeast overgrowth, gas, inflammation and food reactions, plus increasingly poor health, are the result.

Smaller meals help to prevent sugar level ups and downs, ***so you don't crave as much sugar***. Since it's vital for the body to prevent sugar levels from getting too high, it secretes insulin and other hormones to keep our blood sugar levels balanced. The practice of continually eating large meals forces the body to work very hard to control blood sugar levels, eventually wearing out the pancreas, a very serious matter. Eating smaller meals will virtually prevent this.

A note of interest: Numerous researchers have sought reasons why some individuals have lived to the advanced ages of 90, 100 or more and remained in apparently in good health throughout their long lives. These long-lived people came from all ethnic groups, enjoyed a wide variety of occupations and lifestyles, and ate a wide type and variety of foods. Researchers found that there was one primary common denominator that characterized their long lives: They consistently under ate. A lesson to us all.

What shouldn't I eat? In addition to the foregoing information, if in doubt, don't eat it. ***Read labels***; if they contain words you don't understand or can't pronounce, don't buy the product. You'll be better off if you don't. Do your own research, obtain and read some of the resources named at the end of this book. Ultimately, you are responsible for what you eat. ***Become informed***.

Part III

I will praise You, for I am fearfully and wonderfully made (Psalm 139:14).

Understanding Digestion

As pictured below, digestion takes place in a 30-foot long tube that begins with the mouth and ends with the colon. Although the digestive process is far too complex to cover in a publication this size, it's important for everyone to become at least somewhat familiar with the basics. See **Figure 3** below:

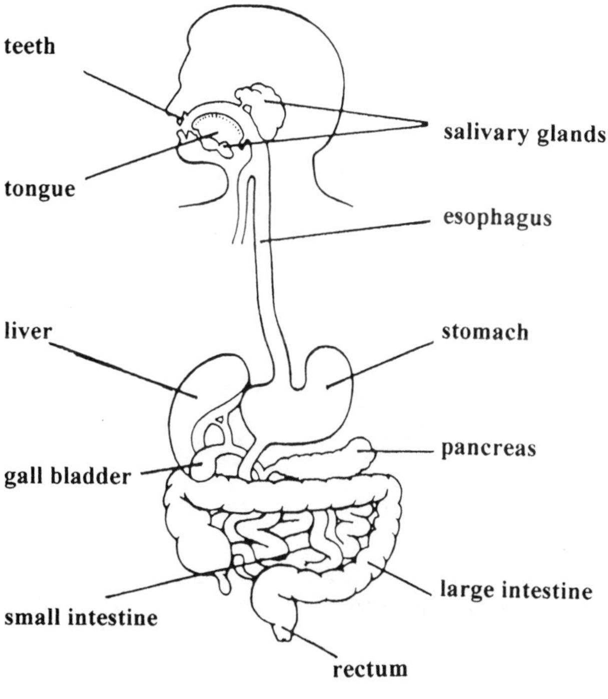

The Mouth

The average person has little awareness or knowledge of either the functions or importance of the **mouth** in the Digestive Process; which is illustrated by the fact that the majority of people suffer from some form of digestive complaint or problem.

1. In fact, the **mouth** plays a very important role in one's digestion, beginning with the moment one bites or places a forkful or spoonful of food into his mouth. But, even before one seats himself or herself at the table (20 or 30 minutes before), ideally, the very first act of digestion is to ***drink a full glass of water***. This will supply the salivary glands (in the oral cavity) with sufficient water to produce saliva and the stomach with sufficient water with which to begin the digestive processes.

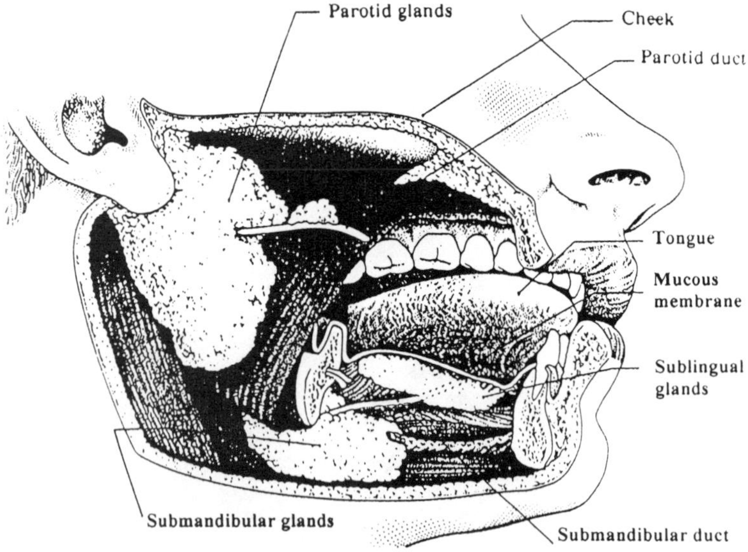

Figure 4. Saliva is so important to digestion that the mouth contains three pairs of salivary glands: parotid, sublingual and submandibular.

2. Then, when food enters the mouth, ***it should be chewed at least 25-30 times for each bite and thoroughly mixed with saliva*** (the body's first-line digestive enzyme). Saliva is a very powerful secretion, with several functions. In addition to its obvious function of mixing with the chewed food, making it ready for swallowing, ***saliva produces lysozymes that attack and destroy bacteria both in the food and in***
3. ***the mouth***; before it is swallowed and passed down the esophagus (food tube) to the . . .

The Stomach

The Stomach's function, as generally understood, is to "digest our food," but, as stated above, digestion begins in the mouth and continues in the stomach.

1. Basically, the stomach receives food from the mouth and esophagus that is (hopefully) thoroughly chewed and mixed with saliva, and further mixes it with hydrochloric acid (HCL), pepsin, water and rennin. HCL and pepsin break down proteins into smaller peptides; rennin curdles milk and dairy products; HCL enhances absorption of iron and calcium; deactivates plant and animal hormones (if food has been chewed properly and thoroughly mixed with saliva); and further kills bacteria!
2. If you are having digestive problems (upset stomach or acid indigestion, heartburn, or burping or belching within a few minutes or an hour or two after eating, you may be one of millions of Americans who are suffering from . . .
3. Hydrochloric acid (HCL) deficiency. Hydrochloric acid is the only acid the body produces and is essential for life. It is the first substance in the stomach that breaks down protein. Without proper levels of hydrochloric acid food becomes a mass of poorly digested acid waste residue. Reduced quantities foretell illness. Note: Salt is necessary to make HCL; totally salt free diets neglect this need.
4. HCL usually starts a disturbing decline around the age of 40, though diminished amounts are found in all ages, even young children. Supplemental HCL will help alleviate al-

most any health problem. If you are having digestive problems, your health professional may suggest the use of supplemental HCL (Betaine Hydrochloride), which can be obtained at most health food stores.

The Small Intestines

The **Small Intestine** is actually an elaborate food processing and waste eliminator plant, responsible for converting foods into an acceptable state for absorption into the body. It constitutes a long (approximately 22 feet) tube of interlooping tissue, connected with the Stomach at one end and the Large Intestine at the other. The functions of the Small Intestine include onward movement of its contents by peristaltic action, secretion of intestinal juices, completion of digestion, protection against infection, secretion of hormones and absorption of nutrient materials.

1. The highly acidified food from the stomach is alkalinized by bicarbonate from the pancreas (without this neutralizing action, the stomach's acid would literally burn holes in the Small Intestine);
2. Where it is mixed with several pancreatic enzymes, along with bile from the liver and gallbladder.
3. The combination of enzymes from the pancreas, the liver and gallbladder, play a major role in digestion.
4. Since our body's production of crucially important pancreatic enzymes declines around the age of 40 (often much sooner), supplemental pancreatic enzymes are usually necessary for optimal digestion.
5. All these enzymes break down food into molecules that are small enough to pass through the wall of the Small Intestines into the blood, where it is distributed to all the cells of the body to be used for energy. The remaining waste matter is moved by peristaltic action into the . . .
6. **large intestines**, where most water is squeezed from the waste matter enabling trillions of bacteria to complete the digestive and eliminative processes.

The Liver/Gallbladder & Pancreas

Though these three are separate organs, the Liver, Gallbladder and Pancreas share a common function: They all send digestive substances to the duodenum (the first section of the Small Intestines) to further the digestive process; although, except for the Gallbladder, this is not their only function. Proper functioning of all three is indispensable in the processes of digestion and absorption. In the illustration below, note how digestive juices from all of these organs converge like tributaries of a river at the common bile duct.

The Liver

If one is to live in Divine Health, it is vitally important to watch over and care for the condition of our **Liver**. This organ is so indispensable to our life, health and well being that God provided it with special powers of regeneration. If, for any reason, our Liver becomes injured or diseased to the point that as much as two-thirds of it is damaged or must be removed, this marvelous organ will completely regenerate itself! Truly an example of Divine healing!

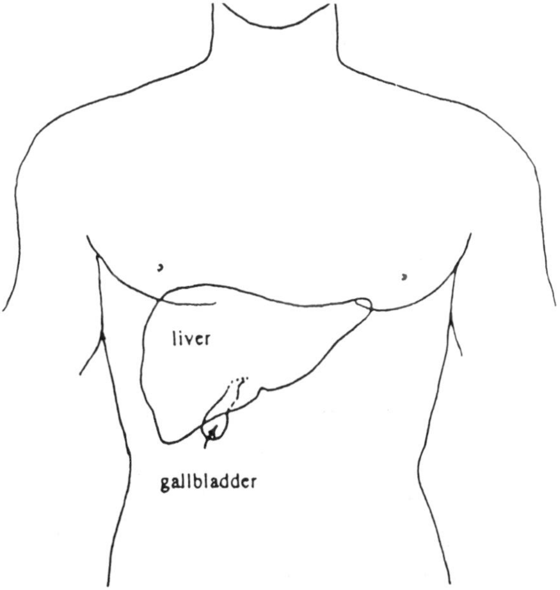

Figure 5. The liver in relation to the gallbladder.

- Weighing between 3 and 4 pounds, and second only to the skin, the Liver is our body's largest organ; body; performing over 500 functions, among them, making (or processing) new chemicals and neutralizing poisons and wastes; and influences the smooth functioning of all our organs.
- As mentioned, it has the ability to regenerate itself in many cases; but ***if the Liver dies, the body dies***. And in every case of compromised health, one's liver function is also impaired in some way or to some degree.
- The chemical genius of the Liver is basic to the strong beat of the heart, wide-open channels of the blood vessels, the soundness of digestion, the sharpness of the brain and the strength of the muscles.
- The Liver secretes a quart or more of bile daily; a greenish liquid, part digestive and part excretory, and sends toxic items along with it to the intestines through the bile ducts.
- Production and elimination of this quart or so of bile each day is a major method of keeping cholesterol levels low.
- Bile is stored and concentrated in the gallbladder; and is essential to the digestion of fats, oils and fat-soluble vitamins.
- If the bile ducts are clogged and an insufficient amount is available in the Small Intestine, the bowel movement will be light brown, or yellow or orange and will float, a clue to bile duct blockage;
- ***You can also expect cholesterol levels to rise, digestion to be impaired and the development of pains throughout your body.*** For example, pain on the right side can come from problems at the ileocecal valve or the appendix, or the large intestine. It can also come from the Liver, which is higher up, but is sending its pain message to your side.
- To clear the clogged bile ducts, you simply do a liver cleanse, over and over, until the problem is gone. This might take several such cleanses, because we have hundreds of larger ducts and thousands of tiny ducts feeding into the larger ones.

- Unless you are ill, you can profit by scheduling a liver cleanse every two weeks until your pain is gone. Remember: A clogged Liver does not necessarily give you pain by itself. It is more likely the bacteria in the gallbladder and bile ducts causing toxic inflammation. (See *Liver Cleanse*, on pages 50-52.)

The Pancreas

The **pancreas** is an integral part of the digestive process. It is a large gland (approximately 5 inches long) situated behind the stomach. The Pancreas is a very busy organ . . .

1. It contains the islets of Langerhans that produce insulin, which helps to balance blood sugar levels and glucagons.
2. It produces pancreatic enzymes, such as pancreatin, trypsin and chymotrypsin that enable the Small Intestine to complete the digestion of proteins. Pancreatic enzymes break down protein wherever it may be found, including ingested protein, parasites and tumors, an action that produces more toxic material, which the liver must deal with.
3. The pancreas also produces bicarbonate to alkalinize the partially digested, very acidic food that flows from the Stomach into the Small Intestine.
4. ***Insufficient pancreatic function is one of the causes for chronic fatigue and lowered resistance.***
5. If you are having difficulty in digesting your food, and are frequently troubled with abdominal discomfort within 2-3 hours after a meal, you might be deficient in pancreatic en-
6. zymes. It would be advisable to ask your health professional to suggest a good source for obtaining supplemental pancreatic enzymes.
7. Note: If you have done the Liver Cleanse described above to improve your health and are also taking pancreatic enzymes, you can help further remove the toxic burden from your liver by doing a coffee enema. (See *The Coffee Enema* on pages 53-55.)

Kidneys

Reddish-brown and bean-shaped, Kidneys are very special organs of elimination (most persons are born with two).

- They filter the body's total blood supply about two times per hour and
- rid the body of toxic substances and other waste products, including nitrogen.
- Additionally, the Kidneys act as Master Chemists for the body; regulate the pH (acid-alkaline) concentration of water balance in the tissues;
- control the balance of sodium and potassium (without which our cells could not produce electrical energy) and
- regulate uric acid levels.
- Kidneys can become clogged with parasites, yeast, fungus, molds, oxalic and uric acid and phosphate crystals (from soft drinks and meats, breads and pastas) and other debris. Kidney stones and otherwise clogged kidneys can affect one's overall health, including the heart and circulatory system, the liver and the brain. By controlling water and salt levels, the kidneys also help control blood pressure. Clogged livers can produce kidney stones.
- If you suspect your kidneys are malfunctioning, you could benefit from doing an herbal kidney cleanse. (See Kidney Cleanse on pages 55-57.)

The Large Intestine

The **Large Intestine** or **Colon** controls the flow of material from the ileum (where it connects with the Small Intestine) the rectum and anal canal or anus. The function of the Colon is to move solid material to the anus for elimination. There are many billions of microbes (both "friendly" and "unfriendly") in the Colon, which help complete the final stages of digestion. Normally these microbes are kept in a healthy, homeostatic balance. However, the overuse of antibiotics will kill all these bacteria indiscriminately, leaving the body's final digestive process in a defective, compromised condition. If antibiotics must be used, it is mandatory that the "friendly" bacteria be replaced as quickly as possible by the use of acidophilus. Lack of attention to this and other bowel problems will ultimately result in a number of other serious conditions that can only be rectified by cleansing the bowel.

Constipation, or an under-active bowel, is a toxic bowel, and will sooner or later host a myriad of compromised-health conditions; because its uneliminated load of toxins will be absorbed through the bowel wall into the bloodstream to be recirculated throughout the entire body, including the brain. The result will be increasing degrees of cell destruction, incomplete digestion, and a downward spiral of energy loss and a weakened, sickening condition.

Obviously, the remedy is to re-activate bowel stasis. Several steps are involved, including improving one's diet, with special attention being paid to ingestion of adequate amounts of water and sufficient high-fiber foods, especially raw, or lightly cooked fresh vegetables and fruits. The next step is to thoroughly cleanse one's colon. (See *Colon Cleanse*, pages 58-59.)

Systemic Toxicity

Remember, unrelieved stress in any form: unforgiveness, hatred, fear, frustration, anger, bitterness, malice, etc., ***act as tourniquets around the heart and blood vessels, including all smooth muscles, nerves, lymphatic system and most organs, affecting every cell in our bodies, and, among other detrimental effects, creates a heavy toxic load.*** Unless one is able to relieve themselves of such toxin-producing stresses, they will eventually result in organ degeneration and sickness.

God's Word counsels us in this regard. We are commanded to "take heed to yourselves, lest your hearts be weighed down with carousing, drunkenness, and ***cares of this life*** . . ." (Luke 21:34). We are urged to get rid of bitterness, rage and anger (Ephesians. 4:31), because such uncontrolled, powerful stressful emotions will weaken us spiritually and make us sick.

Systemic Toxicity is an indication that every cell, tissue, organ and system of the body is toxic. Most of us have thought (or been taught) that when one part of our body is in pain, that only that part of the body is sick. For example, if we have a headache, or backache, we commonly "treat" our head or back, or whatever, with an aspirin or some other pain medication. But, what we haven't considered is this: The pain we feel indicates that a toxic condition exists somewhere in our body, and may or may not be in the particular organ that seems to be manifesting the pain. In other words, pain and a disease condition of any kind is "systemic," meaning a toxic condition exists that is affecting our whole body.

The solution is not necessarily to treat the body with drugs, but to determine the cause(s) of the toxic condition, then to eliminate it. For example, frequently a chronically toxic liver, gallbladder, bowel or other organ will result in systemic toxicity, which, if promptly attended to can avert an acute disease condition. There are many ways to help keep your body healthy and avoid a toxic condition. In the next section detoxification methods are outlined and discussed that will further enable individuals to take responsibility for their own health.

The Thyroid Gland

One might wonder why the Thyroid Gland is included under systemic toxicity, but there is a good reason; largely due to the influence of the late Broda O. Barnes, M.D., Ph.D. Early in his career, Dr. Barnes, in choosing the thyroid gland as the subject for his doctoral thesis, became aware that ***the solution of many of the major health problems*** of the century lies in the "proper care of the thyroid gland: everything from overwhelming fatigue to the really devastating diseases – heart and artery ailments – and, least expected, common emotional disorders, such as depression."

Though Dr. Barnes was a general practitioner, he focused on the thyroid gland, because he believed that its insufficiency and improper function were the unsuspected causes of a host of illnesses. Without his contributions, millions of individuals would today be energyless, living vegetables, old before their time, emotionally disturbed, without understanding why, unable to think or remember (some believing they had Alzheimer's disease), and being treated for symptoms, rather than for the easily correctable, underlying conditions responsible for an estimated 40% of the population. *You may be among that 40 percent.*

The **Thyroid Gland** is a butterfly-shaped organ that appears to wrap itself around our pharynx or throat, and is vitally involved in our energy level. Malfunction of this gland will cause your motor to run sluggishly, resulting in one or more of these conditions: weakness, dry, coarse skin, lethargy, slow speech, swelling of face and eyelids, coldness and cold skin, diminished sweating, thick tongue, coarse hair, pale skin, constipation, weight gain, loss of hair, labored, difficult breathing, swollen feet, hoarseness, loss of appetite, excessive and/or painful menstruation, nervousness, heart palpitations, brittle, ridged nails, slow movement, poor memory, emotional instability, depression, and/or frequent headaches.

If one or several of the above conditions apply to you, you may be one of the one hundred million U.S. citizens who are hypothyroid. What can you do? Your health professional will be able to check your thyroid to determine its normality. However, you can do a simple test yourself, which will give you a fairly accurate idea of your thyroid's function.

Obtain a mercury bulb type oral thermometer. Before going to bed, shake it down below 96°. As soon as you awaken and, before you get out of bed, tuck the thermometer snugly in your armpit for ten minutes while you lie there. Do the test on two consecutive days. If your thyroid level is normal, your temperature should range from 97.8 to 98.2 degrees F. ***If it's lower, you are probably hypothyroid*** (under-functioning thyroid), and your physical problems and related ones have probably been caused or at least influenced by that and you should talk with a health professional about Thytrophin, a Standard Process product.

PART IV

Let us cleanse ourselves from all filthiness of the flesh and spirit (2 Corinthians 7:1).

Detoxification

The following pages include several different methods of strengthening and detoxifying the body. Of course, all of them should not be utilized at once. But over a period of days or weeks, most people will benefit from incorporating one or more into his or her nutritional program.

The Liver Cleanse

The **Liver Cleanse**, which is one of the most powerful procedures you can do to improve your body's health, is not difficult to do. It improves digestion, the basis for your whole health. You can expect some allergies to disappear, more with each cleanse you do. It also helps eliminate shoulder, upper arm and upper back pain. You can also expect more energy and increased sense of well-being.

As stated above, it's the job of the Liver to make bile, 1 to1-1/2 quarts each day. The Liver is full of tubes (biliary tubing) that deliver the bile to one large tube (the common bile duct). The Gallbladder is attached to the common bile duct and acts as a storage reservoir. Eating fat or protein triggers the Gallbladder to squeeze itself empty after about 20 minutes, and the stored bile finishes its way down the common bile duct to the Small Intestine.

For many people, even children, the biliary tubing is choked with gallstones. Some develop allergies, but some have no symptoms. Most gallstones are not visible on X-rays, because most are too small or not yet calcified. As these tiny stones grow and become more numerous, the back pressure on the liver causes it to make less bile. When one's Liver is choked with gallstones, less cholesterol leaves the body, and cholesterol levels may rise. To do a Liver Cleanse you will need:

- 4 tablespoons of Epsom salts
- ½ cup of extra virgin olive oil
- 4-8 capsules of ornithine (an amino acid you can obtain at your health food store)
- a fresh, pink grapefruit (fresh, not frozen)
- a one-pint jar with a lid
- a one-quart jar with a lid

Choose a day, such as Saturday for your cleanse, because you will want to rest the next day. On the day of your cleanse, don't take any vitamins, medicines or any pills you can do without (they could prevent success). **Eat a no-fat and no-oil breakfast and lunch,** such as cooked cereal with fruit, fruit juice, bread and preserves or honey (no butter, cream or milk), baked potato or other vegetables or a salad (no salad dressing) with salt only. This allows the bile to build up and develop pressure in the liver. Higher pressure pushes out more stones.

The schedule: ***Do not eat or drink anything after 2:00 P.M.*** If you do, you could feel quite ill.

- Prepare your Epsom salts. Mix 4 tablespoons in 3 cups of purified water and pour into the quart jar. (This makes 4 servings of ¾ cups each.) Set the jar in the refrigerator.
- **6:00 p.m.** Measure and drink one ¾ cup serving of Epsom salts. If need be, you may rinse your mouth with a mouthful of water.
- **8:00 p.m.** Measure and drink another ¾ cup of Epsom salts. You haven't eaten since 2:00, but you won't feel hungry. The timing is critical for the rest of the program, so don't be more than 10 minutes early or late. Get ready for bed.
- **9:45 p.m.** Measure and pour ½ cup of extra virgin olive oil into your pint jar. Hand squeeze the grapefruit into the measuring cup, removing pulp and seeds with a fork. This should give you ½ to ¾ cup of grapefruit juice. Add to the olive oil, cover with lid and shake until it is watery and

frothy. *Only fresh grapefruit will do this.* Visit the bathroom one or more times, even if it makes you late for your ten o'clock drink. Don't be more that 10-15 minutes late.

- **10:00 p.m**. Drink the olive oil/grapefruit juice mixture. Take 4 ornithine capsules with the first few sips to make sure you will sleep through the night. If it helps you to do so, you may drink through a large plastic straw and/or have a taste of catsup or brown sugar to chase it between sips. *Drink it standing up. Get it down within 5 minutes.*

Lie down immediately. The sooner you lie down the more stones you will get out. As soon as your drink is down lie down flat on your back with your head high on the pillow. Lie perfectly still and try to think about what's happening in your liver. You may even feel a train of stones traveling along the bile duct like marbles. There is no pain because the bile valve ducts are open. Go to sleep.

- Immediately upon awakening in the morning, take your third dose of Epsom salts (**but not before 6:00 a.m.**). If you have indigestion or nausea, wait until it is gone before doing so. You may go back to bed.
- **Two hours later** – take the fourth and last ¾ cup of Epsom salts. Again, if desired, you may go back to bed. After 2 more hours you may eat. Start with fruit juice. Half an hour later eat fruit. One hour later you may eat regular food, but keep it light. By supper you should feel fully recovered.

How Well Did You Do?

Use a flashlight to look for gallstones in the toilet. Look for the green kind; this is proof that they are genuine gallstones, not food residue. Only bile from the liver is pea green. Count them roughly, whether tan or green. Some people will need to cleanse a total of between 2,000 and 3,000 stones before their liver is totally clean. You may repeat this cleanse in two weeks. Never cleanse when you are ill. Congratulations! You have just removed your gallstones without surgery!

The Coffee Enema

Coffee enemas may sound ridiculous, but are more logically beneficial logical than you might at first think. They send a message to the liver for it to release these and other stored poisons, which it then does, resulting in a healthier Liver, and fewer toxic poisons circulating in the blood stream.

- A **coffee enema** is simple to do, but produces great healing benefits. Coffee enemas are not colon cleanses, but are *retention enemas*, enemas that are held in the body for a specified period of time. Unrecognized as a valuable tool by many health professionals, coffee enemas increase enzymatic activity, healthy red blood cell formation and oxygen uptake.
- Coffee enemas work because of a special circulatory system between the sigmoid colon (the very last part of the colon with an "S" curve) and the liver (the Portal Vein or Entero-Hepatic Circulation).

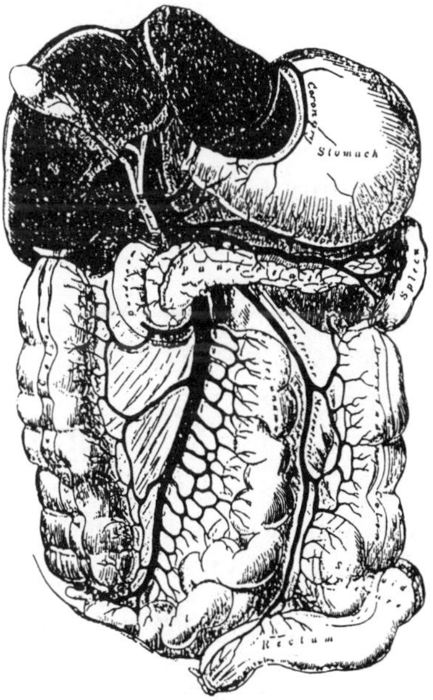

Figure 6.
Entero-hepatic circulation (large, dark blood vessels) carries caffeine from the coffee enema directly to the liver where it becomes a strong detoxicant, causing the liver to dump its accumulated load of toxins, which enables other circulating toxins to then filter into the liver for detoxification.

- By the time the stool gets to this part of the colon, most of all the good vitamins and minerals and other nutrients have been reabsorbed back into the blood stream. But, because the stool is so full of toxins and the products of putrefaction at this point, this special circulatory connection between the colon and the liver sends toxins directly to the liver for detoxification, rather than circulating them through the rest of the body and all its vital organs, including the brain, and making the person sick.
- ***Retention Coffee Enemas*** are an important part of Dr. Max Gerson's cancer program, and Dr. William Donald Kelley used coffee enemas to help cure himself of cancer. Coffee enemas are the best-known cure for headaches. Additionally, a coffee enema makes one feel clean and refreshed. Coffee enemas were regularly suggested by doctors before 1977 when mention of them was removed from the Merck Manual (the doctor's bible of diseases and treatments) to find more room for drug therapies.

The Procedure

1. Put one quart of distilled water in a pan and bring it to a boil, add 2-3 tablespoons of regular grind coffee (not decaffeinated, but preferably organic) and let it boil for five minutes, then let it simmer for 15 minutes. Or, you may make your coffee in a drip coffee maker, following regular directions for strength.
2. Some add one tablespoon of un-sulfured molasses.
3. Cool to body temperature, then strain and pour into an enema bag (obtain this from any drug store).
4. Lay several old towels on the bathroom floor (coffee stains are permanent).
5. Hang the enema bag on the door knob (not the shower head, which is too high). The enema water should flow very gently into the colon. Remember: This is not a high enema or colonic.
6. Lie on the floor and *gently* insert the lubricated (with castor oil or sweet butter) into the rectum 2-3 inches, then release

the enema bag hose clamp and allows the first 1/3 to ½ (2 cups maximum) of coffee to flow in. Stop the flow as soon as there is the slightest amount of discomfort or fullness.

7. Some people prefer lying on their back; others prefer lying on their right side. Either way, it's helpful to gently massage the abdomen during the process.
8. **The goal** is to hold or retain a portion of the enema contents (none to exceed ½ quart) for 10-15 minutes each. Usually 2 or 3 such retentions will empty the bag.
9. ***The purpose is not merely to empty the bag. Holding or retaining, the enema contents for at least 10 minutes each time is your goal.***
10. During that time you may feel or hear a gurgling or squirting out of liquid up under the right rib cage (or directly below your breast bone), which may be your gallbladder or liver discharging its load of toxins into the bowel.
11. Always discontinue the enemas if there is any adverse reaction whatsoever, and discuss it with your health professional at your next appointment.

Suggestion: If you go somewhere and become chemically overloaded and come home with brain fog or a headache, a coffee enema works wonders! Some air travelers have found coffee enemas to be an excellent antidote for jet lag.

The Kidney Cleanse

There are probably dozens of herbs that can dissolve kidney crystals and stones. The following recipe lists several, along with a source to obtain them. If you can obtain only a few of them that are called for, go ahead and do the cleanse anyway. It will just take longer to get the results. The following list of herbs and ingredients, as well as the recipe, have been have used by many people with good results:

- ¼ cup dried hydrangea root. Hydrangea is a common flowering bush.
- ¼ cup gravel root. Gravel root is a wild flower.

- ¼ cup marshmallow root. Marshmallow root is mucilaginous and kills pain.
- 4 bunches fresh parsley (organic if possible). ***Parsley flakes and dried parsley herb do not work.***
- Goldenrod tincture (leave this out if you are allergic to it.)
- Ginger root capsules
- Uva ursi capsules.
- Vegetable glycerin.
- Black cherry concentrate (from health food store or source below).
- Vitamin B6, 250 mg. capsules.
- Magnesium oxide, 300 mg. capsules.

You may order or purchase these herbs from most reliable herb companies, but be careful. All herb companies are not the same. These roots should have a strong, pungent fragrance. If they do not, they will have lost their active ingredients. Only fresh roots can be used. Do not use flakes or powder.

Preparation

1. Measure and set the roots to soak, together in 10 cups of cold purified water, using a non-metal container and a non-metal lid (even a dinner plate will do).
2. After four hours (or overnight) add black cherry, heat to boiling and simmer for 20 minutes.
3. Drink ¼ cup as soon as it is cool enough.
4. Pour the rest through a bamboo strainer into a sterile pint jar (glass) and several freezable containers. Refrigerate the glass jar.
5. After rinsing the fresh parsley, boil it for 3 minutes. Drink ¼ cup when it is cool enough. Refrigerate one pint and freeze one pint. Throw away the parsley.
6. **Dose:** Each morning pour together ¾ cup of the root mixture and ½ cup of the parsley water, filling a large mug.
7. Add 2 tablespoons Black Cherry Concentrate, 20 drops of goldenrod tincture and 1 tablespoon of glycerin.

8. Drink this mixture in divided doses throughout the day. Keep cold. Do not drink it all at once or you will get a stomach ache and feel pressure on your bladder. If your stomach is very sensitive, start on half this dose.
9. Save the roots after the first boiling, storing them in the freezer. When your supply runs low, boil a second time, adding only 6 cups of water and simmer only 10 minutes.
10. You may cook the roots a third time if you wish, but the recipe gets less potent. If your problem is severe, only cook them twice.
11. Also take as directed, but before each meal to avoid burping: Ginger capsules: one with each meal (3 per day).
    Uva Ursi capsules: one with breakfast and 2 with supper.
    Vitamin B6 (250 mg.): one a day.
    Magnesium oxide (300 mg.): one a day.

Some notes about this recipe: This herbal tea, as well as the parsley, can easily spoil. Heat it to boiling every 4th day if it is being stored in the refrigerator; this re-sterilizes it. If you sterilize it in the morning you may take it to work (in a glass container) without refrigeration:

Remember: Vitamin B6 and magnesium can prevent oxalate stones from forming, but only if you stop drinking caffeinated tea. Tea has 15.6 mg. of oxalic acid per cup. A tall glass of iced tea could give you over 20 mg. oxalic acid. Switch to herb teas. Cocoa and chocolate, also have too much oxalic acid to be used as regular beverages. Phosphate crystals are made when you eat too much phosphate. Phosphate levels are high in meats, breads, cereals, pastas and carbonated drinks. Eat/drink less of these. *Drink at least ½ ounce of water for each pound of your weight each day.*

Sources for Herbs (and the bamboo strainer): If you have a reliable source, go ahead and use it. One of the best sources I know is the Self Health Resource Center, 1055 Bay Blvd., Suite A, Chula Vista, CA 91911. (619) 409-9500.

Colon Cleansing

- **Enemas:** Colon cleansing may be accomplished by self-administered enemas, which flush the lower intestines. Substances generally used in an enema include, water, coffee, herbal tea, mild soap solution, wheat grass juice, oil or another nutritional substance. Always take some form of acidophilus, yogurt, buttermilk or kefir afterward, to replace natural bacteria of the colon.
- **Colonics:** "high enemas" administered by colon therapists, using special equipment to clean the entire colon. Many people prefer colonics to self-administered enemas or clay-and-fiber cleanse described below. All these methods can be helpful to help empty the colon of uneliminated matter. Professional Colonicists can be found in the Yellow Pages of your telephone directory.
- **Colema:** In conjunction with a short fast, described in detail by Dr. Bernard Jensen (*Tissue Cleansing Through Bowel Management*), this process uses a Colema Board, a safe and easy way to take a high enema. If your local health food provider does not carry colema boards you may obtain one through HOPE Foundation: (818) 365-4202.
- **Clay and Fiber Cleanse:** A colon cleanse composed of a fibrous material and clay that can remove years of accumulated, caked-on materials from the walls of both the small and large intestines. If left to accumulate, this caked-on material interferes with the absorption of nutrients by the bowel. *Psyllium* is a good fibrous material to use , in conjunction with *bentonite* or another clay solution (both of which can be purchased from a local health store).

1. The psyllium attracts moisture into the bowel, improving bowel function. The moisture causes the psyllium to expand, filling the intestine. As it passes through the intestines, it drags out the stored waste not ordinarily excreted.
2. The clay absorbs toxins and helps carry them out of the colon. Not more than three such clay-and-fiber cleanses

should be done in a year, with at least two months between them.

Preparation:

1. Mix 1 tablespoon of the liquid bentonite solution in a pint jar with 4 ounces of tolerated water.
2. Add 1 tablespoon of psyllium husks. Cover and shake well. Drink the above mixture quickly after you shake it. The longer it stands, the more it will clump. Drink this mixture three times a day, between meals for 3-4 days.
3. Take no food two hours before or for two hours afterward. Drink at least eight, 8-ounce glasses of water a day (more is better). Since this mixture can be constipating, you might also do a plain water or coffee enema each day.

Some people feel abdominal discomfort the first day or two of the cleanse when the psyllium has expanded in the bowel. Many people pass various particles and substances of varying size and shape. Some report long casings that may be mucosal debris and dead cells covering the surface of the intestinal walls. The colon cleanse will also remove organisms from the gut. This helps reduce the level of unwanted bacteria, yeast and parasites. Be sure and take acidophilus for at least five days after your colon cleanse.

IN A PERFECT WORLD . . .

there would be no pain, no sickness, no disease and no suffering. There would be no clouds of pollution hanging over our cities, nor loads of toxic waste buried in our deserts or dumped into rivers and streams already clogged with sludge and refuse.

The air surrounding our planet and the waters lapping its shores would be pristine: clean and free of smog and acid waste. Neither plant nor animal, fish nor fowl, nor the peoples of the land would be choked or sickened by the fouled food and water given to them for nourishment.

But, today's environment is not perfect. It has been polluted by Man: the very epitome of God's creative power. Instead of the health and well-being our Creator intended for His people, we find ourselves struggling to maintain a measure of health

Our bodies were not created to ingest and to survive on the offal of man's destructive "progress."

What is there for us to do?

Jesus told us to "occupy" till He shall come. God told us to take care of the world He created for us.

"And the Lord God took the man and put him in the Garden of Eden to tend and guard and keep it" (Genesis 2:15, Amplifed Bible). ***To tend and guard and to keep . . .***

What does it mean "to occupy and tend and guard and keep?"

Personally, we believe that "to occupy" includes God's purposes: tending and guarding and keeping the God-created and God-furnished foods He provided for us. And to honor God by carefully caring for and nourishing these wonderful bodies He gave us.

> *Do you not know that your body is a temple of the Holy Spirit, who is in you, whom you have received from God? You are not your own; you were bought with a price. Therefore, honor God with your body (I Corinthians 6:19-20, New International Version).*

It is our prayer that the information furnished in this book will provide you with the knowledge of how our bodies are constructed and how they function, and do so in a way that will enable you to pray for your health and healing more specifically than ever before. And that you will be able to cleanse and nourish your body more faithfully and surely than before.

And that in so doing you will attain, regain and/or retain the health and healing that you seek.

May the Creator of our wonderful bodies
heal you and keep you in Divine Health.
Shalom.

Suggested Personal Research Reading

Elvis Ali, N.D., *ADD & Hyper-Activity,* ***AGES*** Publications.
Elvis Ali, N.D., *The Tree Tea Bible,* ***AGES*** Publications.
Elvis Ali, N.D., *Natural Remedies and Supplements,* ***AGES.***
Nancy Appleton, Ph.D., *Lick the Sugar Habit,* Avery Publishing.
Dr. Theodore A. Baroody, Jr., *Alkalize or Die,* Eclectic Press.
Batmanghelidj, F., M.D., Your Body's Many CRIES for Water.
Hulda Clark, Ph.D., N.D., The Cure for All Diseases.
William Dufty, Sugar Blues, Warner Books Inc
Udo Erasmus,BS.c., Ph.D., Fats that Heal, Fats that Kill.
Mary Ellen Hettinger, Home Remedies from the Bible, Globe Com., 6401 NW Broken Sound Blvd., Boca Raton, FL 33487
Bernard Jensen, D.C., *Tissue Cleansing Through Bowel Management, From Simple to the Ultimate.*
Jacqueline Krohn, M.D., **Frances A. Taylor, M.A.., Jinger, LMT,** *Natural Detoxification,* Hartley & Marks.
Stephen E. Langer, M.D. and James F. Scheer, *Solved: The Riddle of Illness.*
C.S. Lovett, *Jesus Wants You Well!,* Personal Christianity.
Gary Null and Steven Null, *How To Get Rid of the Poisons in Your Body,* Simon & Schuster.
Bob L. Owen, Ph.D., D.Sc., C.R., *Dr. Anne's Cancer Journal.*
Bob L. Owen, Ph.D., D.Sc., C.R., *Roger's Recovery from AIDS.*
Bob L. Owen, Ph.D., D.Sc., C.R., *You Don't Have To Die Sick.*
J. D. Ratcliff, *Your Body & How it Works,* Reader's Digest Press.
Sherry A. Rogers, M.D., *No More Heartburn, Stop the Pain in 30 Days – Naturally.*
Ray Sahelian, M.D. and Donna Gates, The Stevia Cookbook.
Strong's Exhaustive Concordance *of the Bible,* Nelson Publishers.
Martin Teitel, Ph.D., & Kimberly A. Wilson, *Genetically Engineered Food: Changing the Nature of Nature.*
Lorna R. Vanderhaeghe & Patricia J.D. Bouic, Ph.D., The Immune System Cure, Optimize Your Immune System in 30 Days.
Andrew Weil, M.D., Spontaneous Healing and 8 Weeks to Optimum Health

Dear Drs. Bob and Elvis . . .

Dear Dr. Bob, not until I read your books did I fully realize the active role I must take in my own health and healing. I had just assumed that all I had to do was to pray for God to bless my health, regardless of what I put into my body. How very wrong I was. Thank you for helping to open my eyes. God bless you.
Pastor Glen, Tennessee

Dear Dr. Elvis, Thank you for helping me and my family to start living a healthier and natural life and educating us about naturopathic medicine.
Ashmeed, Trinidad and Tobago

Dear Dr. Bob, what a difference you have made in my life. Your patient and kind guidance over the years has enabled me to use your down-to-earth knowledge of nutrition to help both myself and to pass it on to help others. I look forward to many years of good health. My prayers are with you always.
Dorothy, Canada

Dear Dr. Elvis, we at Sangster's Health Centres want to thank you for your devotion to people's health. It is because of people like you that the public is learning to take better care of themselves.
Roy Sangster, Canada

Dear Dr. Bob, thank you for speaking at our church. Your message was encouraging and made an impact on our people. I heard several comments from people about how your message inspired them ***Pastor Philip, California***

Thank you, Dr. Bob, for the nutritional advice you gave me and my husband. As a result, Tom has fully recovered and is back at work again. Your books and counsel are very valuable and much, much appreciated. God bless you. We're eternally grateful.
Helen, Minnesota

Dear Dr. Bob, though I have never met you personally, your telephone counsel has blessed our entire family. My prayer is that God will use you and your wise knowledge to help bring health and healing to many more. Shalom!

Michael, South Carolina

Dear Dr. Bob, your telephone call undoubtedly saved my life. You made me both fully aware of the desperate condition I was in, and also directed me on the pathway to life and regained health. I thank you with all my heart. God bless you always!

Barbara, Washington

Dear Dr. Bob, enclosed is a gift to enable H.O.P.E. Foundation to help some others. Your advice and services are invaluable. Best personal acclaim. ***Grant, Canada***

Dear Dr. Elvis, Assalam Alaikum . . . Thank you for your kindness and may Allah continue to bless you on your journey beyond optimum wellness. *Hazrah and Hakim, Toronto, Canada*

Dear Dr. Bob, thank you for all of your help. My parents and I all feel better knowing that I'm finding ways to take steps toward health. You are much admired and appreciated.

Gina, Oregon

Dear Dr. Bob, thanks for sharing your expertise with us. In your presence I feel God. You are a pure spirit. I love your commitment to people; to health. You radiate both health and love.

Jann, Canada

Dear Dr. Bob, you really are a very special man and we feel the Lord has brought you into our lives. We are here to support you and help to share in your mission. Love and prayers.

Bob & Winnie, Washington

Dear Dr. Bob, as I set about the work of healing, I am deeply grateful for your ongoing help in providing distilled information

and walking me through the labyrinth of terms of medical meanings. Also I take note of the patience you exert . . . knowing so much, but having to wait until those you love are ready to hear and learn what you have to say. You are indeed a great man with an expansive spirit and deepening, ever-expanding mind.

Mary Anne, Oregon

Dear Dr. Elvis, you are a great inspiration and we greatly appreciate your help in naturopathic medicine.

Shaliza, Trinidad and Tobago

Dear Dr. Bob, you somehow seem to keep constantly on the cutting edge of natural ways to keep yourself and others healthy. Your commitment to health is an inspiration to Barbara and me as we continue to help others to live healthily. *Clint, Nevada*

Dear Dr. Bob, the natural healing methods you brought to my congregation and me has blessed us. We all look forward to having you present for another Wellness Seminar.

Pastor Doug, California

Dear Dr. Elvis, we look forward to your seminars and all our staff wishes you continued success in educating West Indians in holistic medicine.

Zerena, Trinidad and Tobago

This is a sampling of the many communications we receive from those who are receiving and putting into practice the message of health and healing from H.O.P.E. Foundation (Health Offered People Everywhere). If you would like to receive information concerning our tapes and books, or to invite Dr. Bob to speak at your meeting, or if you are unable to locate an alternative health professional, and believe you could benefit from a counseling session with Dr. Bob Owen (by phone or in person), you may contact us at H.O.P.E. Foundation. P.O. Box 10600, Mission Hills, CA, (818) 365-4202 / FAX (818) 365-4803.